The Agony

Anne felt something explode inside her head! Her eyes locked onto the spiral-shaped overhead light fixture, where writhing snakes began pouring out from around the rim of its dish-like structure. She watched in unbelief as the metal fixture uncoiled from the ceiling in one powerful thrust, transforming itself into a whirling corkscrew that drove swiftly downward and struck directly into her face with enough force to annihilate her. She was left in perfect darkness. It was ended!

Jan. 26, 2001

To Elizabeth Williams,

With thanks for a wonderful visit to our house.

Malcolm Mac Gregor

The Ecstasy

She felt herself stretched out on her back along the narrow rim of a large eight-foot wheel that extended down into the floor, and which turned slowly underneath her. Her head was thrown back, hanging down along the curve of the rim, her mouth open in pure abandon. The voluptuous sensations spilled over her and increased with the turnings of the wheel. The doctor called out her name and asked her to look into the mirror that had been strategically placed for her to witness the birth. She replied with difficulty, "I cannot. It is too much!" She made an effort to lift her head, but it fell back again in ecstasy.

The Miracle

After the nurse left the room, we resumed our new-found EMT pain-controlling technique. Again it worked perfectly. As long as the endorphins were stimulated, the brain did not interpret the nerve impulses from the laboring uterus as pain signals. Anne lay comfortably on the bed, with no sign of any serious discomfort. We continued on in this manner for another two hours. Finally, the nurse appeared again. Since she had heard nothing at all from our room, she hadn't intruded on us during those two hours. But now it was time to make another check on Anne's progress. The nurse lifted Anne's hospital gown and peered under. "Oh, my God," she exclaimed, "You're ready to deliver!"

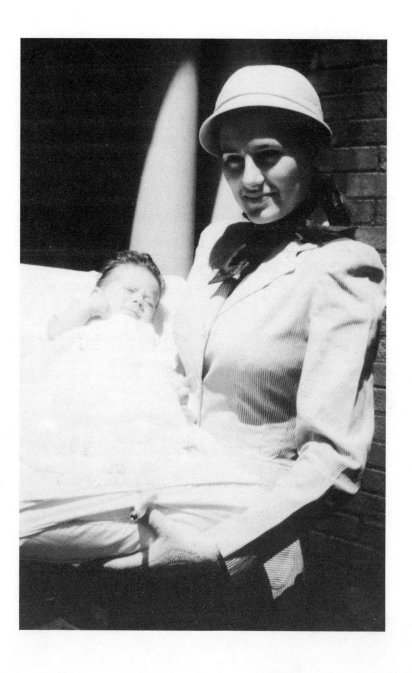

The Agony
The Ecstasy
The Miracle

Three True Childbirth Stories

*Three stories, told from the viewpoint of
the husband, that could change our
attitude toward childbirth*

J. Cameron, Ph.D.

The Agony   The Ecstasy   The Miracle
Three True Childbirth Stories

El Mac Books
P. O. Box 3300
Livermore, CA 94550
U.S.A.

Printed in U.S.A. by Wesley H. Turner, Printing
Cover design by Josh Gitomer

ISBN 1-886838-03-8

Library of Congress Catalogue Card Number: 95-60074

First Printing 1995

1 3 5 7 9 8 6 4 2

Table of Contents

Frontispiece

The photograph shown on the frontispiece, and also on the front cover, is a picture of my wife Anne and our first son. It was taken in front of our apartment building, three weeks after his birth. Anne had the birth experiences described in the three stories that make up this book. The trauma she went through while giving birth to our first son is described in detail in *The First Childbirth Story*. The beautiful exterior Anne exhibits in the picture conceals the chaos this childbirth created within her. Her lifelong struggle to overcome her inner turmoil is a truly moving example of the power of the indomitable human spirit.

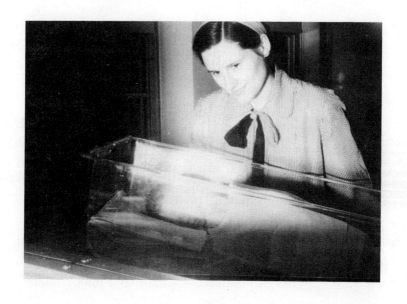

This picture shows Anne with our first son, who is in his baby bed in the nursery, immediately adjacent to her hospital room. It was taken just before they were discharged from the hospital, six days after the delivery. The reflected glare from the flashbulb unfortunately obscures the view of the baby.

What You Can Learn From This Book

The first Childbirth Story described in this book happened to my wife, and indirectly to me, more than forty years ago, in just the way it is presented here. The second occurred about three years later, and the third twelve years after that. The reason I am finally writing them down is that these experiences may be of help to couples who are now facing the prospect of childbirth. The first Story, which is the longest in the telling, is a tale of medical teaching gone wrong; of unwitting and unnecessary physical and emotional damage inflicted on an expectant mother in her time of travail. The second Story forms a brief vignette that describes a marvelous mystical orgasmic birth experience which some doctors know about, but which they usually do not care to discuss with their patients. The third and final Story, which is also in the form of a brief vignette, tells of a remarkable discovery my wife and I stumbled upon accidentally, perhaps uniquely. This fascinating discovery constitutes the main *raison d'être* for the present book. It opens up an unsuspected prospect for less painful childbirth. If you read nothing else in this book, you should read the final pages that make up this third Story. Because the discovery revealed there has been limited to just my wife and myself, and in only a single occurrence, its universality is open to question and to further investigation. Hopefully, the present book will help to stimulate research into the possibilities of this technique.

These are intensely personal stories. They contain the kind of information that one does not commonly discuss with one's friends, or even one's family. The stories relate to the childbirth process itself, which, apart from the death process, is probably the most universal of the important events that shape people's lives. One would think that, given the advances of the twentieth century, modern medicine must have thoroughly explored all of the avenues which are of importance in this singular event, but this is not the case. Nature's plan for the design of the mechanism that brings babies into the world still contains unanticipated surprises.

About the Author, His Wife, and His Book

My work is science. I have a Ph.D. in physics, and I have published many research papers and two books during my professional career. Anne is my wife of almost half a century. She has an M.A. in art. In her early twenties she worked as an interior decorator. Then she raised a family, and now she is a painter and sculptor.

The idea for this book occurred to me as I was reflecting on our early years as young parents. I was struck with the realization that Anne's three childbirth experiences were unique and deserve to be told. Together, they form three related stories. The first story is a lesson in how *not* to conduct childbirth. The second and third stories open up new and largely unexplored avenues for extending the scope of the childbirth experience.

Each of the events described here occurred thirty or more years ago, and no one, apart from a few psychiatrists and other medical doctors, has ever been told about them. Even our children haven't heard them.

I have written these stories in such a way that they do not reveal the names of the people involved, nor the locations or precise times where the various events took place. But they are not fictional. Every event that is portrayed here, down to the smallest nuance, is given exactly as Anne and I remember it. I haven't made up anything. Some events in our lives fade away and are forgotten. But the events described here were so dramatic and unusual that they have been forever stamped into our memories. I am writing them down in the hope that the lessons they teach will survive after my wife and I have passed on.

The First Childbirth Story

The Agony

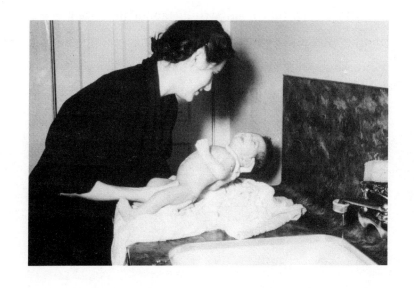

Anne is shown giving our new son a bath in the kitchen sink in our upstairs apartment. He was about two weeks old.

18

A Prologue to Disaster

The events that I am writing about here took place many years ago. Time has dimmed my recollections of some of the memories, but the main events were burned in so indelibly that they did not fade away, nor did the feelings associated with them. Anne and I were each twenty five years old at the time of this first childbirth. Looking back from my present perspective, those were tender years, with the vicissitudes of life still lurking unexpectedly around the corner.

It was a bright spring morning when Anne and I entered the front door of the massive teaching hospital and wended our way to the maternity ward. Her pregnancy had been absolutely normal and uneventful. In fact, she had worked at her job as an interior decorator right up to the very day the doctor had predicted for her delivery, and there had been a large office party that evening to celebrate her departure for the imminent duties of motherhood. However, two weeks then elapsed before the signal finally came that the time had arrived, and we were now somewhat nervously checking in at the hospital for this momentous new experience of birth and parenthood.

We didn't really know what to expect, but we seemed to be in the best of possible hands. The hospital prided itself on being one of the finest institutions of medicine in the country, and our personal physician was no less than the august Professor of Obstetrics himself. How could we do better than that? We were about to receive the best medical care during childbirth that modern science could render. We had prepared ourselves by reading Dr. Grantly Dick-Read's pioneering book *Childbirth Without Fear*. (This book was loaned to us by one of the student nurses at the hospital, the wife of a friend of mine.) Anne had followed the recommended exercises laid out in the book, but with no encouragement from the medical community, who in those days felt that childbirth was a procedure best left in the hands of the physicians. We came armed with a cribbage board, which we planned to use to while away any spare hours before the baby was born. And we were armed with the naiveté of the young and inexperienced.

Little did we suspect that two and a half days later my wife's life, and hence my own, would be irrevocably changed. In that sixty-hour period, her physical and mental health was dealt a blow from which it has never fully recovered. During the forty-odd years that have passed since that experience, there probably hasn't been a single week in which I haven't at some time or other silently cursed the memory of the Professor of Obstetrics. To give the Professor his due, he was a sincere and dedicated medical man, and he never realized to his dying day, a few years later of leukemia, that during my wife's delivery he had violated the first tenet of his Hippocratic Oath, which goes roughly as follows: "Thou shalt not act in such a way as to bring harm to thy patient."

Before embarking on this story, let me first supply some background information about my wife, who is the protagonist, the one who experienced these events, and also about myself. My role in this story was mainly limited to that of an occasional observer and, now, of chronicler.

Our Early Years

Anne (her parents called her Anna) was born in a Polish community in a large midwestern town, and English was her second language. Her parents were both born in Poland. She was the fourth of five children. Her family suffered through the turmoil of the Great Depression. Life, for immigrants with little education and only a poor proficiency in English, was a constant financial struggle. For survival, there were times when the community soup kitchen provided the evening meal. The family home was on the West Side, in a poor neighborhood where ethnic issues were very much in evidence.

Anne first attended a Catholic parochial school, where the lessons were taught in Polish by Polish nuns. She was a bright pupil, a slender tow-headed little girl with a big smile and the nickname "Sunshine." Later on, she transferred to a public school, an "English school," where she was double-promoted to a higher grade level. She had a flair for music and learned to play the guitar, which was almost as large as she was. At a young age, she appeared as a regular performer on a Polish Hour program at a local radio station, accompanying herself on the guitar as she sang folk songs.

During high school Anne did a lot of the family housework, because both her mother and father were employed. There was no time left over for participation in high school sports and extracurricular activities, though she yearned for such experiences. When World War II came along, her older brothers and older sister all enlisted in the Armed Forces. After graduating from high school, Anne won a typing and shorthand competition, and thereby obtained a job as a secretary at the army depot in town.

Anne grew up in a working class neighborhood. Although there were many bright students among the immigrant population, none of them considered going to college. The young men graduated from high school, went into the service during the war, and then took industrial jobs with the various companies in town, rarely moving away from the area. The women, not all of whom graduated from high school, worked for a while at clerical or secretarial jobs, got married early, and started raising families. Anne was an exception to this scenario.

She decided early on that she would get a college education, no matter what obstacles stood in her way. Her parents had no money to support her ambitions, and they themselves had only the briefest of educations in America. Her mother had come to America at the age of one, and she was the third eldest of thirteen children, all of whom started to work at early ages. Her father had come over from Poland at the age of fourteen, and, although he could barely speak English, had served in the cavalry in the American Army during World War I, where his early training with horses stood him in good stead. His three older brothers, one of them a Catholic priest, all died of pneumonia in the great flu epidemic that swept through America and the world in 1918.

Anne worked for a year after graduating from high school, and then, at the advice of an "English" friend of hers, applied for a scholarship at the private Protestant university where her friend was a student. Even though she was Catholic, she was awarded a scholarship to this university, where she concentrated on Spanish, with the idea of going to South America as an English teacher. She also took courses in art. In her freshman year, she went out for the drama club, and she became the first freshman in the school's history to be given the leading role in their annual play. She was also one of the four co-eds selected together as the campus beauty queens.

After two years her money gave out, and Anne had to drop out of school and return home and go to work. She started as an assistant in a furniture store, apprenticed herself to the store's interior decorator, and quickly learned the trade. Her flair for color and design was apparent, and she soon had clients of her own among the wealthier families in town. She also attended school part-time at a nearby Catholic college. The following summer she took a week's vacation, met me, and changed the course of her life.

My early years were in some respects similar to Anne's, and in some respects very different. They were similar in that we both had immigrant parents. Anne's parents spoke English with a Polish accent. My mother was born in Hungary, and at age fourteen came to America by herself, just before World War I. She spoke English with a Hungarian accent. My father was born in Canada, and thus was not really a "foreigner" in the ethnic sense. My mother had come to America to live with her uncle, who died shortly after she got here. She was taken in by a caring American family, who helped her to obtain a couple of years of high school education. She later supported herself as a hairdresser. My father graduated from high school in midwestern Canada, taught at a small one-room school in western Canada for four years, and returned home to help on the family farm. He then put himself through university, where he obtained a degree in chemistry and, at age thirty two, was captain of the soccer team. He moved to the United States, obtained a job with a chemical company, and met and married my mother. I was born a year later, and two brothers followed afterward. My father was fortunate enough to retain his job all through the depression, but the threat of a layoff hung over his head the entire time, just as it did for all of our neighbors. He worked for twenty years at the same salary, and was glad to have it.

In grade school, I learned to play the piano, as did my brothers. I can remember going around to various PTA meetings at a young age and playing for the assembled parents. In high school, I was a good student and was class president. I went out for the debate team in my sophomore year, and we got to the quarterfinals in the state. I played in four varsity sports, lettered in three of them, and did none of them very well. Halfway through my senior year, I volunteered for the navy in order to stay out of the army. My eighteenth birthday was spent in a navy bootcamp.

Two years later World War II ended, and I held the ranking of Aviation Electronics Technicians Mate First Class. I had spent one year in radio technician school and then one year teaching radar navigation. I never got overseas. During this time, I decided I would go into physics. As soon as I was discharged, I enrolled in college, majoring in mathematics and physics. Later I obtained a summer job as the radio technician on a university research project in a wilderness area, met Anne, and succeeded in persuading her that we should share our future together.

After we met, Anne decided to return to university for another year of schooling. I continued on with my studies, obtaining a degree in mathematics the following spring. In September, Anne and I were married, and we set up housekeeping in a second-floor apartment in an old building attached to a drug store on the edge of the campus. I had now entered graduate school in physics, which included a Teaching Assistantship to help pay the bills. Anne obtained a job as an interior decorator in an exclusive decorating studio in town. It was a very prestigious job, although it didn't pay a large salary. We started out with orange crate furniture, while Anne was at the same time decorating some of the swankiest homes in the area. She was twenty three years old.

After a year of marriage, Anne became pregnant with our first child. I still had several years of graduate school ahead of me. We decided that she would work as long as she could, and then she would become a home-maker, possibly working on some limited part-time basis after the baby's arrival. We knew several student nurses at the University, and one of them recommended the Professor of Obstetrics as the best man to have for our doctor. The choice seemed unassailable, and we were able to enlist his services. Anne's pregnancy was absolutely normal. She worked all the way through, having none of the ills sometimes associated with pregnancy, and she looked forward to motherhood with a great deal of anticipation.

One thing that is perhaps of importance here is the deferential attitude which Anne and I had towards doctors at that time. In the communities where we had been raised, the few college graduates we knew personally were mostly teachers, and the people who had obtained post-graduate education were limited to doctors and dentists. In those days, the doctor was a man of high status, both professionally and economically, and his opinion on any medical subject was taken as law. The dictates of the doctor were followed unhesitatingly. Thus, when a doctor told us something, it never occurred to either of us to question it. Forty years later, we have quite different opinions on this subject, but this is knowledge born of rather painful hindsight. Doctors are mere mortals, like the rest of us, and the best of them make mistakes. The judgment of the doctor must always be considered carefully, but the judgment of the patient, who has a greater vested interest, is also of importance. In cases where doubt exists, a wise patient is well-advised to trust his own instincts. But it takes time to learn these things.

It is against this background that our story really begins.

The First Forty Eight Hours:
Much Ado About Nothing

It was a Wednesday morning when we entered the University Hospital. The birth of the baby had originally been expected two weeks earlier, but the signals were only now directing us to the hospital. Anne had had occasional contractions for a few days, but they were now coming at frequent intervals, every fifteen minutes or so. When she called his office, the Professor told Anne to pack her suitcase and come to the hospital.

For its day, the hospital was rather advanced in its handling of childbirth. Fathers were allowed into the labor room with the mother, which was not generally the case in most hospitals. But they were not allowed to be in the delivery room. And the doctors were not yet interested in any of the "natural childbirth" exercises which were just starting to come into vogue. As to anesthesia, the Professor of Obstetrics in this hospital customarily used a "saddle block" (caudal) while delivering the baby. This was administered into the lower spine, near the end of labor, and it deadened all sensation in the lower part of the body. We knew these facts, and they were about all that we did know about the practical aspects of the childbirth process.

In addition to her personal belongings, Anne had packed a cribbage board, so that we could play a few games if the time seemed to be dragging along. As it turned out, we had plenty of time to play. After we entered the hospital and were directed to the labor ward, Anne was assigned to a labor room and "prepped" by a nurse. I then joined her. There were several labor rooms in the complex, and we could hear when other couples were coming or leaving.

The morning passed uneventfully. The contractions did not start building up to anything, but neither did they stop enough to warrant Anne's being sent home again. We played a game of cribbage, which Anne won. Although I pride myself on my skillful play, she always seemed to inexplicably turn out to be the winner, and this time was no exception.

Lunch time arrived, we ate, and the afternoon came along. We were vaguely aware from the various sounds in the hall that someone had left the labor ward for the delivery room. There followed another cribbage game, and an idling away of the time. In medical circles, the mucus plug that emerges when the bag of waters surrounding the baby is broken is known as the "show." Anne and I made up some lighthearted jokes about "Let's get this show on the road."

Dinner time came and went. We were aware that one or two others had entered the labor ward. The contractions were still continuing pretty much as they were when we first entered the hospital. During her pregnancy, Anne and I had studied the material in Dick-Read's *Childbirth Without Fear.* She had practiced the prescribed breathing exercises, and I had tried to become proficient in my role as her support system during labor. As I recall it now, this consisted in large part of massaging her lower back during the contractions and trying to help her relax. The main idea behind the breathing exercises was to lift the stomach wall away from the uterus. With each new contraction, Anne and I did our best to follow the recommended procedures, but they didn't seem to make much difference. The contractions themselves were not particularly painful at this stage of the proceedings, but they had the unfortunate effect of keeping Anne awake and full of nervous anticipation. The Professor popped in occasionally to have a look, but he had no advice to give us, and he showed no interest in my supportive measures.

Evening turned into night. Some of the light-heartedness we felt about this adventure was beginning to fade. It didn't help our confidence any that during the time we were there, other expectant mothers had entered and left the labor ward. We seemed to be making no progress. All through the night and into the next morning we kept each other company, at times with little jokes, and at other times just in silent waiting.

Finally it was time for breakfast. Anne and I were both a little bleary-eyed. We weren't used to this kind of sleep deprivation. Neither of us had slept a wink. The contractions seemed to be going on endlessly, not with any really uncomfortable intensity, but not with any effective results either. The second day passed just like the first. Other eager and expectant couples came into and left the labor ward. We seemed to be its only long-term occupants. Another game of cribbage was played, but our enthusiasm for it had waned. I was still practicing back-rubbing, which had no effect at all. Lunch came, then dinner, and the situation went on as before. Our jokes about "getting the show on the road" now possessed an irony they had not had before. Student interns and student nurses appeared from time to time, but they had no advice to offer. They were learning, just like we were.

Another long night passed. The contractions continued on and picked up somewhat in intensity, so there was no sleep for either of us, but they didn't seem to be leading anywhere. The enormous bulge that Anne carried in front of her made it clear that there was indeed a baby there to be born, but it didn't seem to be in any hurry to come out. By morning we were both totally fatigued, not having slept for two days and two nights. The Professor came around and assessed the situation. He suggested that my presence in the labor room didn't seem to be helping things, and he advised me to go home and get some sleep. He told Anne to go and take a shower.

Our two days in the labor room had produced no tangible results. What it had done was exhaust Anne at a time when she needed all of her strength for the ordeal that still lay ahead. She, of course, did not know what this ordeal was to be, nor did I. It was perhaps just as well that we didn't know.

The Next Ten Hours: Lonely Pain Without Progress

I went home, tumbled into bed, and slept like a log for about four hours; then I roused myself, dressed, and headed back to the hospital. When word was passed to the maternity ward that I was coming in, a young student intern quickly came to the entrance. "You aren't allowed to be with your wife," he said. "The Professor has left instructions that you are not to see her."

"How is she doing?" I asked.

I don't remember his answer, but it was something to the effect that nothing much had changed. He stood there with the obvious intent of making sure that I didn't try to enter the labor ward. Had I attained my present maturity, I would have insisted on seeing Anne to ascertain for myself what was going on. But in those days I didn't question the authority of anyone I saw in a white coat. I left the hospital, took a long walk along the banks of the nearby river, and cried. I can remember looking up at the windows of the hospital and wondering which one opened onto the room where she was laboring away.

Anne told me later that she had spent most of the day by herself in the labor room. Young interns entered from time to time. They examined her for signs of progress, and then entered their findings on a large blackboard at the main desk which recorded the most current data on all of the mothers laboring in the complex. The problem was that Anne wasn't dilating, even though the contractions were now quite vigorous.

In late afternoon, I was sitting in the waiting room of the maternity ward when the Professor appeared and said I could now see Anne. He told me that she had been laboring all day long, and that the contractions were strong, but she just couldn't relax and let go. "She's all tied up inside," he said. I remember thinking that maybe he should be taking some responsibility about helping her to relax, but I didn't say anything. He obviously felt that helping her to relax was not a part of his role as her obstetrician. Then, right out of the blue, the Professor looked directly at me and said something which struck me as unusual. He said, "You'd like to have those contractions for her." That statement could well be true, but it certainly didn't tie in with anything he and I had ever discussed. In light of what happened later on, it may have told more about him than it did about me.

When I entered Anne's room, I saw her for the first time in the throes of the real pangs of childbirth. As a contraction came on, she cried out and sobbed. She looked very pale and tired. She had been laboring in this manner all day. The Professor took me outside of her room and advised me that he intended to burst the bag of waters as a way of speeding up the labor. I stood outside by the door as he entered her room to do this. There was a short period of absolute silence, and then a heartrending scream. I remember thinking to myself that the Professor seemed to have the bedside manner of a "truck driver." He hadn't said a thing to Anne to cushion her for what he was about to do. After he emerged, carrying a stainless steel bed pan with a cover on it, I went into her room. Anne was vomiting into a tray held by a student nurse. I noticed that Anne's lower abdomen was completely distended. Her bladder had filled up during the course of the day, and the pressure of the baby had blocked the urethra. This had finally come to the attention of the Professor, and he had instructed the nurse to insert a catheter. I don't know how it feels to have a bladder that distended, but it didn't look like something I would care to experience. And how must it feel when the baby's head presses against it during a contraction? Anne did get one moment of satisfaction here. She told me that after the bag of waters had been ruptured, she looked into the bed pan, saw the large mucus plug we had been waiting for, and knew that "the show was on its way."

The Professor next told me that he was going to give Anne a sedative to put her to sleep for a while. "She is completely exhausted," he said. The sedative was administered, and then Anne and I were left alone in her room. For perhaps an hour and a half we were quietly in there together. Anne was feeling no pain. She wasn't really asleep, but was in sort of a twilight zone. If I said something, she would answer me, but her voice was very detached. I felt very close to her, and very concerned for her well-being. I also felt very helpless. We husbands may be necessary for starting the baby in the first place, but as potential fathers, we are (or at least were at that time) accorded a very limited role to play when the baby is being born.

Finally Anne was making signs that she was coming out of the sedation. The Professor appeared and said that I would have to leave her room and stay in the hospital waiting room. I did not realize when I left that the next time I saw Anne, she would be a different person. When I returned to Anne's room, I was two hours older, and Anne was twenty years older.

The Final Two Hours: Descent into Darkness

In spite of John Donne's famous poem, it is a fact that in many respects each person is an island unto himself. We share some experiences, but some things we go through are known only to the person involved. My experiences during the next two hours were as different as they possibly could be from the experiences Anne had during those same two hours.

As instructed by the Professor, I went out to the maternity ward waiting room. Anne seemed to be doing all right when I left her (she was still coming out of the sedation), and I was hopeful that things would somehow proceed in a reasonable manner. There were several men and women in the waiting room, and we engaged in pleasant conversations about various childbirth and hospital stories. One topic that came up was how long people stayed in the hospital after childbirth. The University Hospital where our story took place was at that time typically keeping the post-partum mothers and their babies in the hospital for seven days. However, the mothers were gotten out of bed on the first day after birth to look after their babies, which in each case were kept in a nursery adjacent to the mother's room. Thus the new mothers were by no means bed-ridden for those seven days. One lady in the waiting room was an older person who had had children many years earlier. She said that in her day, she had been kept in bed in the hospital for two weeks after the birth, and was then taken home on a stretcher. And this was after a perfectly normal delivery! We all commented on how times have changed. As of this writing, the time in the hospital for most new mothers and their babies has been cut down to a day or so after normal deliveries. Hospital procedures continue to change.

After about two hours, a nurse appeared and informed me that Anne was ready for the delivery room, and that I could come and see her for a minute. When I went in, she was on a gurney and ready to be wheeled to the delivery room. There were two or three young interns in white coats standing around, and they looked at me rather curiously as I entered. I didn't think much of it at the time, but later on, when I learned the story of what had gone on in my absence, this circumstance took on a lot more meaning. I can't remember exactly how Anne looked, only that she was very quiet as she lay on the gurney. I took her hand and wished her luck in the delivery room. Then she was wheeled off. That was all I knew about those fateful two hours.

It was weeks and months before I learned from Anne what had gone on while I sat peacefully in the waiting room, talking with the other expectant fathers and relatives. And the story I finally pieced together is one that even today causes me to wake up in the middle of the night and rail at the injustice in the world, at the damage inflicted on innocent people.

Although Anne had described to me various events that occurred during her childbirth, we had never put the pieces of information together to see the whole picture. When, more than forty years later, I made the decision to write this book, I asked Anne to sit down beside me and tell me everything that had happened. She still recalls the whole experience very clearly, and many of the things she told me were things I was hearing for the first time. I have endeavored to reproduce her account of those final two hours, at least the parts where she was conscious enough to remember.

This next paragraph is speculation on my part, but in view of subsequent events, I am sure it is essentially accurate in its main suppositions.

The Professor had a pretty good idea of just what to expect when Anne came out of the drugged semi-sleep into which he had placed her. She had had at least some semblance of rest, and her uterus had also received some cessation from its efforts. So it would begin the contractions with renewed vigor. Since the bag of waters had now been ruptured, the contractions would become more effective in dilating the cervix. Thus Anne would be moving rapidly into second-stage labor, which in reality is the most painful part of the birth process. Furthermore, Anne had already received considerable medication, so the Professor would have to be careful in giving her additional sedation. But the Professor had more than just the patient on his mind. It was his duty, as he saw it, to expose his obstetrics trainees to the full panoply of childbirth experiences, including the sight of a patient in intense pain. They were going to have to deal with these situations later on, and they had better know how to evaluate them. This seemed to be a good opportunity for them to observe a patient in the final stages of labor, and he didn't intend to pass it up. He alerted his medical students to be ready to come into the labor room when he gave the word. Subconsciously, the fact that Anne was a very beautiful young lady and would make an attractive centerpiece for his exhibition may have also been a factor in his plans, although he would never admit that, even to himself. And, of course, the last thing the Professor wanted was to have me floating around and gumming up his plans. So I was firmly escorted to the waiting room when the time came.

As I have stated, the above scenario is speculation on my part, since I was not privy to the Professor's innermost thoughts. But what happened after I left Anne to go to the waiting room is a matter of public record, which is to say, it is a part of Anne's recollections. After I had been safely tucked away out of sight in the waiting room, the Professor called his staff of trainees into Anne's room. Anne was lying on a twin-size hospital bed, with the head of the bed against the wall. Approximately ten young student doctors and nurses "in training" crowded into the small room and arranged themselves along the sides of her bed, right next to the bedrails that had been raised on either side. (Anne told me that until she saw the manuscript I had written for this book, it never occurred to her that these people were *students*. She had assumed they were regular medical staff. In fact, it concerned her that so many doctors were present. Was something wrong?) By placing himself at the foot of the bed, the Professor assumed his role as the teacher in a classroom. The group was silent. No one spoke. Anne was still groggily struggling back into consciousness. The contractions were occurring steadily and strongly. As they crested, she cried out in pain. The student doctors and student nurses pressed closer, intent on observing her behavior.

Anne's uterus, refreshed by its sedated rest, now intensified its efforts. Anne said that at this point she could no longer distinguish individual contractions. Instead, there seemed to be a steady grinding and churning in her abdomen that went ceaselessly on and on, giving her no respite from her labor—no time in which to recover between onslaughts.

The force of the contractions increased even more, and now Anne no longer had a choice in her reactions. The intense pain from the contractions, added to her fatigue from the ordeal of the past sixty hours, and the bewildering after-effects of the drugs, stripped away any remaining restraints. Her defenses crumbled. Anne was completely out of control. She writhed in agony on the bed, screaming for help at the top of her lungs. As the pain rose to its highest pitch, Anne reached above her head and frantically took hold of the metal bars at the head of the bed. She repeatedly jammed her head against the bars as she tried desperately to withdraw from the fire in her belly. But there was nowhere to exit!

Anne told me that when the pain in her abdomen reached the point where it had become one long uninterrupted torment, the passage of time ceased to exist. Time no longer had any meaning for her. We normally experience time as a sequence of events that occur one after the other in a linear chain. But Anne no longer recognized such a chain of events. For her there was only *one event* —an unendurable agony that surrounded and engulfed her, and it wasn't going anywhere. With her mind riveted to her belly, she was unable to think about anything else. In telling me about it, Anne could recall all the details of her suffering, but she had no idea how long it lasted. She had no time frame in which to structure her experiences.

Time did not move as slowly for the students gathered around the bed as it did for Anne. The students were here for a purpose. The Professor was teaching a lesson. We can imagine his message: "It may be difficult for you to stand here and watch this, but this is an important part of your training. Soon you will be doctors and nurses, and then you will be in charge of your patients. If a patient of yours is going through a crisis that is unpleasant to watch, you can't simply go away and return when it is over. You have to stay and see the crisis through. You have to be able to witness any kind of a crisis and still keep your composure, like I do. That is why I have brought you together here." The Professor didn't say these words out loud. He didn't have to. The students understood.

For perhaps an hour, the demonstration that the Professor had orchestrated in the labor room dragged on. Anne lay agonizing on the bed. All the while, she was "boxed in" on three sides by the Professor and his students. The room was brightly lit for the occasion by a ceiling fixture which was located over the foot of the bed. This enabled the students looking down on Anne from their positions next to the bed to see clearly every detail of her torment. From Anne's viewpoint, looking up at them, the world appeared as a frame of white inert coats illuminated by a merciless white light. During her ongoing ordeal, Anne was acutely aware that the doctor who was "in charge" was in fact not in touch with the human part of her. The Professor stood there the whole time, silently observing Anne. What his thoughts were, we will never know.

The only sounds in the room came from Anne as her abdomen contracted and convulsed with its efforts to send forth the baby. To Anne, that hour must have seemed an eternity. Spurred on by the incessant, unbearable cramping in her womb, she continued screaming without letup—straining again and again against the metal frame at the head of the bed. Anne's innermost soul was laid bare for all to see and hear. We can only wonder what damage this searing public exposure inflicted on her innate sense of privacy, her dignity, her self-esteem.

How much pain can a laboring woman endure? This depends to a considerable extent on her physical condition. Anne's physical condition had been excellent when she first entered the hospital, but now, *sixty hours later*, it was not. Apart from an hour and a half of drugged sleep, she had not slept at all during that time. She had had only minimum amounts of food, and some of that had been vomited away. She also had minimum amounts of water, and the process of laboring had forced some of that out, as evidenced by her distended bladder in the late afternoon. Vomiting also contributes to dehydration, which can be a major problem during an extended labor.

On top of all that, we can only imagine how much the frenzied thrashings of the past hour had taken out of her. Physically, Anne was now spent.

Anne was also mentally and emotionally exhausted. She had been in a painful phase of labor for twelve hours, and she wasn't getting anywhere. There was no sign of progress. The torment just went on and on. Finally, an inconceivable thought forced itself on her: *there is no baby!* This thought had a certain logic to it. If nothing is coming forth, maybe it is because nothing is there. Though the thought was very persistent, Anne was aware that it contradicted what she *knew*: there *was* a baby in her belly. As she argued with herself over the impossibility of this thought, she realized that she was starting to lose her contact with reality. She desperately needed a reassuring human touch, a touch that would maintain her connection with reality.

Turning to a young student doctor standing at the right side of the bed, Anne held up her hand to him. "Will you please take my hand?" she pleaded, looking directly into his eyes. To her surprise, he made no response. He did not even acknowledge that she had

spoken. She then turned to a young student nurse standing at the left side of the bed and held up her other hand.
"Please hold my hand?" Again, there was no response.
The student doctor and student nurse were keenly aware
of the presence of the Professor at the foot of the bed. He
had arranged this spectacle, and he did not want any of
his students interfering with it. He was calling the shots.

The Professor, without speaking, made it very clear
to his students that they were not to involve themselves
emotionally. If he had wanted them to take hold of
Anne's extended hand, he would have signaled his ap-
proval. *He did not.* The Professor had chosen this time to
teach his students another lesson. He was answering the
question we posed above: how much pain can a laboring
woman endure? His answer was non-verbal, so we can
guess along with his students as to its content: "You
young people don't have the experience in these things
that I have. You have stood here for the past hour and lis-
tened to this young lady screaming her head off in total
loss of control. You have watched her writhe and squirm
all over the bed. You think she is going out of her mind
from the pain, and you wonder what you should do about
it. Well, you should do exactly what I am doing. You

don't have to do anything at all. These women are incredibly tough. She will get through this all right, and she will be just fine afterwards." Unfortunately, the Professor was terribly, tragically wrong.

Anne looked wildly around at that sea of frozen faces. A stunning realization forced itself on her: "These people aren't allowed to express human feeling. They aren't allowed to touch or comfort me. They aren't going to do anything to help me stay connected to reality." As this realization penetrated her understanding, Anne was flooded with a feeling of total despair. She told me later, "I felt I was totally abandoned." She realized that there was going to be no human support—no anchor to reality. There was going to be no human voice speaking to her, no one to sympathize with her, to give her guidance, to tell her that her baby would finally get born. There was going to be nothing, nothing at all, not even privacy in which to suffer alone.

Faced with the chilling prospect of total isolation, Anne was gripped in a wave of panic and bottomless fear which swept over her. At that precise moment it happened!

Anne felt something explode inside her head! Her eyes locked onto the spiral-shaped overhead light fixture, where writhing snakes began pouring out from around the rim of its dish-like structure. She watched in unbelief as the metal fixture uncoiled from the ceiling in one powerful thrust, transforming itself into a whirling corkscrew that drove swiftly downward and struck directly into her face with enough force to annihilate her. She was left in perfect darkness. It was ended!

Anne's brain had, for the moment at least, ceased all normal response to the situation at hand. Anne thought later that she had temporarily lost consciousness. As she explained it, "I stopped struggling. I think I went limp." From that point on, she remembers almost nothing.

Anne never told the Professor about this explosion inside her head, and he never realized what he had done to his patient. It wasn't until many years later that a surgeon-turned-psychiatrist, who was thoroughly familiar with her experiences, ventured to explain to her, and to me, precisely what had happened. "In moments of absolute terror," he said, "the blood pressure can get extremely high. That explosion inside your head was a stroke." Then he looked at her sadly and said, "That's not the way we practice medicine." It was clear that, in his opinion, the stroke should never have been allowed to happen.

The description of the sensations and thoughts Anne had when the stroke occurred is accurate. The words above are based on her recollections. Today, more than forty years later, Anne still carries the pictures of her experience intact. She recalls some of her specific thoughts, as for example: *there is no baby!* This was not a trivial idea. Anne said it had an enormous impact on her. The thought increased in intensity until it was like a "neon sign" (her description) insistently forcing its message on her. (A few days after her delivery, Anne had told me about having this thought, but I did not at the time appreciate its psychological significance. Unable to cope any longer with the unending flood of pain signals, *her brain was starting to construct its own version of reality.* Anne instinctively recognized this, which is why she finally appealed to her silent audience for reassurance.) Anne demonstrated for me how she held up her right hand for help.

She recalls the remote looks on the faces of the students who rejected her pleadings. She even drew me a sketch of the overhead light fixture, which she says is so common that she has since seen it in other hospital and commercial settings. The explosion inside Anne's head and the incident of the snakes squirming out of the light fixture are events that were described to me not long after her delivery. But the story of the fixture leaping down on her and the details of her subsequent loss of memory are things I hadn't heard about until I started writing this book. Anne still relives both her terror and her amazement as she tells the story of how the fixture rammed her face. "Once it happened," she recalls, "I was finished. I was out of it!"

What did the Professor and his students observe at the time of Anne's stroke? We don't know. Nothing was ever reported to Anne or to me. The Professor never said a word about Anne passing out, or exhibiting unusual behavior. If Anne did in fact suffer a physical and emotional collapse in front of a room full of students right after being turned down in her pleas for assistance, this might be something the Professor would not care to admit to us. He might not even want to enter it into the medical record.

Anne's contractions evidently continued on through all of this, because a little while later she was dilated and ready to deliver. She has no recollection of caudal being administered. Anne remembers being told at some point that she was ready for the delivery room, but she cannot connect it to other events.

Finally the hoped-for event happened! The contractions did their job—the cervix was opened. This is one of the most intensely painful stages of the birth process. What was Anne's reaction to it? She doesn't remember. Sometime after her stroke, Anne must have returned to conscious awareness. I base this on the fact that she was conscious—but very subdued—when I saw her on the gurney before she went into the delivery room. A few weeks after the delivery, Anne informed me that the only thing she heard the Professor say during the entire time she labored in front of his students was his terse comment that she was now ready for the delivery room. Her next statement to me was one which I still clearly remember, but which she no longer recalls: "When he said that," she told me, "I shut up." Evidently some part of her remembered her persistent screaming.

Anne was wheeled into the delivery room, and was there for an hour. She has only one brief mental picture from that entire period, which she later described to me:

She remembers herself lying on her back, probably on a gurney, in a large cold room filled with many varied pieces of metal medical equipment. Because there was no sound, she at first thought the room was empty. Then, when she turned her head to the left, she saw in a transparent plastic box, about twelve feet away, a baby. She reasoned that it was her baby. She remembers wondering why he was a grayish color instead of pink. (She didn't know that babies have to be cleaned up after birth.) In spite of her exhausted state, she yearned to hold him, to see him up close. But after embracing him with her eyes, she seemed to lose consciousness again.

This is the totality of Anne's memories in the delivery room. She remembers no details of the birth.

The good news from all of this was that Anne delivered a perfect eight and a half pound baby boy. The bad news was that Anne emerged a shattered wreck. Life from then on was never to be the same again. Nine years of psychoanalysis was not sufficient to undo the horror of that experience.

What can we say about the behavior of the Professor in all of this? He was an honorable man, well respected in his profession, and a man who worked long and hard to tend to his patients. But this does not mean that he was without blame, without an obsessive interest in some phases of the birth process. I learned from a student nurse at the University that the Professor had a habit, which seemed to be unique with him, of insisting on a vaginal examination in each of his patients two days after delivery. The nurse commented that these vaginal examinations were more painful than the delivery itself. The degree of rapport between the Professor and his patients can perhaps be ascertained by the rapport between the Professor and his own wife. He monitored her fourth pregnancy, took care of her at the hospital during labor, delivered her himself, sewed up her episiotomy after the delivery, and only at that point realized he was about to become the father of twins!

What can we say about the behavior of the students? For an hour they stood beside a woman in extreme agony and made no effort to relate to her in a human way. In fact, following the example of the Professor, they psychologically kept their distance. This is what he was training them to do. Anne was not a laboring mother in distress, but rather a clinical subject for observation. In this teaching situation, the students really had no choice in their actions. The fault lay with the Professor. The fault would not be with the students unless and until they went forth and taught others to act in this same manner.

The demonstration that the Professor had arranged for his students only partially conveyed to them the realities of childbirth. As the students filed into Anne's room, they could not have anticipated they were about to participate in an activity that would inflict permanent physical and psychological damage on a suffering human being. Incredibly, after they had filed back out of the room, none of them probably realized they had done just that. And neither did the Professor!

This story of Anne's ordeal unfolded more than forty years ago. Thus we might expect that the science of obstetrics has advanced a long way since then, which it probably has. But some things do not change! In a recent alumni magazine from this same university, I read an article in which the writer complained that the obstetricians at the University Hospital seem to be showing an undue interest in the sufferings of their patients. The teachings of the Professor, long since deceased, may have carried on to the present time! One can only wonder how many other Annes have had their quality of life needlessly ruined by inhumane obstetrical practices.

I once read an article about the tactics the Nazi Gestapo used to "break" their victims. Three steps in the process were listed: *first*, the normal living habits of the victim were disrupted, as for example by sleep or food deprivation; *second*, the victim was worked over late at night, when the body spirit is at its lowest ebb; *third*, the idea was conveyed to the victim, while under torture, that he was in a totally isolated situation wherein no one else knew of his predicament, and no one was going to come to his rescue. He was given to understand that the unbearable pain he was enduring was going to continue on and on. The Gestapo agents were well aware of the importance of psychological factors in the breaking of the human spirit. During Anne's childbirth experience, all three of these factors were present. The first two factors, the sleep deprivation and the birth late in the evening, were of course not under the control of the Professor. They just happened to work out that way. The third factor, however, the psychological factor of complete isolation, with no help forthcoming and no promise of an end to the torment, was completely in the Professor's power to control. He could hardly have acted in a more inhumane manner than he did. And he "broke" his patient. The Freudian psychoanalyst who subsequently spent nine years trying to help Anne cope with her problems said the medical treatment she received at the University Hospital was "criminal."

Dr. Grantly Dick-Read pioneered many of the humane concepts which have now become part of modern obstetrical practice. He recognized the ravages that can befall a woman who has undergone an unbearably painful childbirth. Warnings to this effect are spread throughout his book *Childbirth Without Fear*. Dick-Read's book is a perpetual best-seller, and is currently available in

Harper Paperbacks, Harper Collins Publishers, New York, Fifth Edition. On page 224, Dr. Dick-Read wrote the following:

"The scars of physical pain do more to ruin a woman's life, her marriage, and her motherhood than is generally recognized. It is necessary for a woman to have a scar from a cesarean section, ... but I would rather see the scar tissue of safe healing than the evidence of brain tissue incurably damaged by the shock of pain and terror."

Dr. Dick-Read was a prophet ahead of his times. His contemporaries were hostile to his ideas. Discouraged by their opposition, he tried to burn his first manuscript, but it was rescued from the flames by his wife. Pressured by the British medical profession, he moved his medical practice from England to South Africa. At the time of Anne's first childbirth, obstetricians in general were not nearly as concerned as Dr. Dick-Read was about the emotional dangers of childbirth trauma. The Professor clearly shared the general view.

The Troubled Aftermath

The obstetrical staff at the University Hospital did not at that time encourage new mothers to nurse their babies. They preferred to have the babies put on bottles. In fact, there was even talk of cases in which unsuspecting new mothers were given "drying-up" medicine against their wishes. But Anne was determined to nurse her newborn son. The nurses did not permit her to do this on the first day after the delivery. Instead, she was given bottles of sugared water to feed to him. It wasn't until the second day, thirty six hours after the delivery, that she was allowed to put him to her breast. By that time her breasts were completely engorged and feverish from the pressure of the trapped milk. In her subsequent childbirths, the baby was brought to her much earlier to nurse.

The University Hospital was an experimental "lying-in" hospital. Under this arrangement, new babies were kept in small nurseries next to the mothers' rooms (see the picture on page 12), and nurses taught the new mothers how to care for their babies. The first day after the delivery, Anne was kept on her feet much of the day learning to clean, diaper, and feed her baby. The second day also. On the third day a sign was hung on her door, "Do Not Disturb." She had caved in from the overload of the entire experience. A few days later she arrived home with our new son, and our life as parents began.

Our second floor apartment consisted of a couple of rooms in one of the city's oldest houses. Indeed, on a recent visit there, we discovered that it is now designated as an historical building. The living conditions in this old house were not well-suited for the task of raising a new baby. In the wintertime, the community steam heat was turned off every evening at ten o'clock, and a thick layer of frost formed on the insides of the window panes during the night. Since disposable diapers did not exist at that time, and we had no laundry facilities, we were dependent on a nearby laundromat. Also, my being a graduate student did not fit in well with the role of fatherhood. Nor did the fact that my prelims in physics were scheduled a month after the baby was born. Passing these exams was *the* essential requirement for acceptance as a Ph.D. candidate. Being totally dedicated to furthering my career in physics, Anne made every effort to ensure my success. I still recall the many evenings she stood wearily at the kitchen sink (the one shown on page 18), washing dishes or diapers while I studied. Somehow we got through that month. Seven of us took the preliminary examinations. I was one of the three who passed. But the victory had its price. Anne's first month as a nursing mother was not the pleasant experience it should have been.

The ravages that had happened to Anne as a result of her childbirth trauma only gradually became apparent. Unfortunately, we had read about the "post-partum blues" in a book on childbirth. A little learning is a dangerous thing. It kept us from realizing sooner than we did that Anne was in trouble. According to this book, it was normal for a new mother to feel tired and depressed. Thus when Anne felt this way, it seemed to us that it was only to be expected. However, after a few months it began to dawn on us that perhaps something more serious had occurred.

Anne desperately wanted to continue nursing the baby. But at a routine checkup visit to the Professor three months later, she told him she was so totally exhausted that she would have to stop. He agreed. He didn't inquire as to why she was so tired, or why she had lost so much weight. It should be noted here that our third child, born fourteen years later, was nursed by Anne for nineteen months.

The effects of a stroke are difficult to assess, especially when the stroke is not even diagnosed. A massive stroke can cause paralysis or even death. That obviously did not occur here. Anne could do everything she had done before, but she couldn't do things as well or as easily. After a few months Anne went back to work one day a week as a decorator, because we needed the money. Before the birth, she had been able to perform complex business calculations at the studio without effort. Now, she could still do the mathematics, but it seemed to be a lot harder, and she made mistakes. Whereas before she had been able to glance through books and pick out the relevant information almost as if by osmosis, now reading was an effort. The secretary at the decorating studio said that Anne's footsteps didn't sound like her any more. She had lost her natural ebullience. She used to skip along, and now she sort of shuffled. When her handwriting before the birth was compared with her handwriting six months later, it looked like the writings came from two different people.

There were physiological effects from the trauma. Anne's arms and legs seemed to ache all the time, for no apparent reason. A doctor gave her one kind of muscle relaxant, then another, and then a third. None of them helped. The most obvious problem was an overwhelming sense of fatigue. Months after the delivery, Anne would lie in bed during the day for hours on end in a sort of a semi-stupor, with the baby in a crib beside her. The sleep she got during the night brought no refreshment. Her vitality, which had been her trademark, was gone.

Perhaps the most insidious effects were psychological. Recent Pavlovian experiments on animals have shown that when a fear response is imparted to the brain of an animal, it cannot be erased, and it does not fade away. The fear response can be partially overlaid with a more benign imprint, but its effect cannot be completely masked. During Anne's childbirth experience, she had been exposed to moments of abject terror, and this trauma disturbed her mind at the deepest subconscious level, where it could never be dislodged. After the birth, Anne found that if she was left totally by herself, with no other adults around, she would sometimes experience a nameless fear that came out of nowhere and preyed on her. She would call me up at my school office and ask me to come home and reassure her. There was one terrible occasion when I was working on my thesis research late at night in the locked physics building, and Anne had a sudden panic attack. She was unable to reach me by phone. Leaving the baby unattended in his crib (which is something she would *never* do under normal circumstances), she put her coat on over her night clothes and ran the several blocks from our apartment on the edge of the campus to the physics building. It was Fall, and the night was raw and windy, which is probably one reason why she had felt so lonely in our apartment. As she ran along the campus sidewalk, a branch from a giant elm tree broke off and crashed directly in front of her path. Had it fallen two seconds later, our story would have had a different ending. As she approached the physics building, Anne could see the light on in the third floor laboratory where I worked. It was well after midnight, and mine was the only light on in the building. Anne picked up some pebbles from the ground and tried to get my attention by hurling them at the lighted window. But she couldn't throw them high enough (see the picture on page 77). I never realized that she was there. She finally went home and toughed it out alone. After I got back, very late that night, and saw her, I swore to myself that I would never put her in that situation again.

Another panic attack occurred when Anne was home on a Saturday morning. I was again at the physics building. (I was always at the physics building.) Anne phoned me and said that I had to come and take her out to see people. "I have to see some people," she said, "Anyone." I came and got her and the baby, and we walked to a nearby coffee shop. As it happened, the doctor who was now her physician (the one who gave her the muscle relaxants for her aching limbs) was also in the coffee shop. I explained to him why we were there. He was very surprised. He could see her obvious distress. "Does she often act like this?" he asked. He never pursued this matter any farther, either then or when he subsequently saw Anne in his office. This doctor was currently serving as the head of the local Catholic hospital, so he clearly was a competent physician. He had been recommended to us by another member of the University Hospital faculty. But I don't think he understood Anne's situation at all. As a matter of record, Anne had never shown the slightest sign of any kind of problem like this before childbirth. And yet none of the doctors in that town who saw Anne as a patient ever suggested to us that her trauma in childbirth might be responsible for her problems.

After the childbirth, Anne started having trouble sleeping at night (and still does). If she got into an "overload" situation, everything would seem to completely break down. A sudden noise or disturbance could trigger a violent startled reaction in her. Once, just before we departed from the University after my graduation, Anne went to a psychiatrist at the University Hospital for an evaluation of her problems. He said she was "a fertile field for schizophrenia."

How long do these traumatic imprints on the brain actually last? There were times, thirty years later, when I would wake up in the middle of the night to find Anne, who was in the throes of depression because of another sleepless night, sobbing softly to herself, "They wouldn't take my hand." These imprints can last a lifetime.

This is not the only memory from Anne's crisis that remains embedded within her. Years later, she would be lying tensely next to me in bed, and she would say, "Please tell me that everything is going to be all right." I would take her in my arms, and I would say, "Anne, everything is going to be all right." Then, as if a switch had been thrown, she would suddenly relax. She just needed to hear this reassurance spoken out loud. During her crisis, there had been no one there to tell her this.

Prolonged human suffering penetrates deep into the psyche. But there is a difference between just prolonged physical pain, as in the case of a broken leg, and the kind of suffering which, together with the pain, includes mental and emotional trauma. When simple physical pain is unbearable, we try to steel ourselves against it. We endure it because we know the sickness or wound will heal. When the pain stops, we tend to forget what it was like. But when psychological factors are a part of the trauma, standing up to the pain becomes almost impossible. In Anne's case, psychological factors contributed to her collapse. As a child, Anne never saw a doctor, except on one occasion when she had a strep throat infection. Her family couldn't afford doctors. From her earliest years, whenever Anne had a "hurt" of any kind, her mother would lay her hand on it, and it would go away. Her mother was never too busy to pay attention to her, and she never acted as if the hurt wasn't important. Anne was conditioned to regard human touch as comforting—even healing. In view of this, it is not surprising that when Anne was in her deepest crisis in childbirth, when she felt her contact with reality slipping away from the relentless onslaught of the pain, she turned to the one thing that *she knew would save her*—a human hand holding hers. When this was denied her—not once but twice—it was the final straw that broke her spirit.

The psychological stress that Anne sustained had one final devastating consequence—her loss of "self." When people are in unendurable pain, their most private behavior is wrested out of them, and they are doubly shamed if others are there to witness it. The protective shell that surrounds them is torn away. For this to happen in an intimate personal situation is bad enough. For it to happen in public, on a brightly-lit stage, without permission or forewarning, is a frightening invasion of privacy. The victim feels violated, psychologically cheapened. Being rejected by a *group* of people carries with it a special kind of weight. Group disapproval carries a finality, like a verdict given by society: we will not acknowledge you—you do not exist. That is what happened to Anne. She could never again face people with the same sense of self-assurance that she had shown before the baby was born. She often expressed her confusion and frustration by saying, "I'm not myself. I've lost my identity. I don't seem to have a sense for picking out a dress for myself anymore." I have heard her say a hundred times, "I'm just not *me*."

Dr. Grantly Dick-Read, more than anyone else, is responsible for the support systems which are available to laboring women today. The point he clearly recognized was that a first-time mother requires constant emotional reassurance. He particularly stressed the role of the husband in providing this, and he emphasized the need for pre-natal instruction. In his book *Childbirth Without Fear*, he commented again and again on the extreme psychological vulnerability of an anxious woman in her first childbirth. On page 242, Dr. Dick-Read wrote the following:

"... no patient should ever be left alone. No greater curse can fall upon a young woman whose first labor has begun than the crime of enforced loneliness. Why cannot every obstetrician realize the enormity of this medieval torture."

During Anne's long ordeal, I was with her for her first forty eight hours. But of course I really knew nothing about the childbirth process. My fumbling efforts at back-rubbing may have been more of a hindrance than a help to Anne. The really crucial hours in Anne's labor were her next ten hours. The uterus had finally started to contract with more vigor, and she was for the first time in real pain. I had assumed that since I wasn't allowed to see her during this period, someone on the staff was taking my place in looking after her. But it didn't happen that way. Most of the time Anne was left alone! The medical trainees who came in periodically to examine her showed no personal interest. They didn't appreciate her emotional concerns or her physical exhaustion, and they seemed to know little about important factors such as hunger, dehydration, and the necessity of keeping her bladder emptied. All they really checked on was how much she was dilating. This is precisely the situation that Dr. Dick-Read was attempting to warn us about. Filled with anxiety, Anne made no progress in her labor. Her anxiety used up the remainder of her physical and emotional strength. When I saw the Professor at the end of this ten hour period, he said that Anne was spent and had not accomplished much. But he didn't say why. I can't help but wonder how Anne would have fared if she had had an understanding obstetrician such as Dr. Dick-Read in attendance during this fateful time.

The *loneliness* that Anne experienced during her ten hours of "pain without progress" was nothing compared to the *isolation* she felt during the final two excruciating hours of her labor, when she was surrounded by an aloof crowd of observers who wouldn't even speak to her, much less hold her hand. This total withholding of any emotional support at all during Anne's time of crisis is accurately characterized by Dr. Dick-Read as "medieval torture," and it occurred at one of the most "advanced" twentieth-century medical centers in the world. From a psychological point of view, Anne's first childbirth could not possibly have been handled more ineptly than it was.

The Professor had known Anne during the pre-natal period *before* her first childbirth, and he still treated her afterward. Yet he never noticed, or at least never let on to us, that he saw any change in her at all. He was an obstetrician and gynecologist, and his interest in his patients was mainly limited to just the reproductive system.

It took two more years after prelims for me to finish my degree. This included the time required to write my thesis. I can still see Anne, pregnant with our second child, sitting at the typewriter wearing only a slip in the sweltering summer heat of our apartment, typing on the manuscript. It was seven years since I enrolled at the university, and four years since our marriage.

After graduate school, my new job took us far away from the University, and from our families. Anne finally sought psychiatric help, because none of her problems seemed to be clearing up. For nine years a Freudian psychoanalyst struggled with her to try and unearth all of the hidden time bombs and defuse them. The analysis helped, but it didn't succeed in restoring her to her original state of health. Even Freud couldn't put Humpty Dumpty together again. I also spent several years in Freudian analysis, trying to ascertain my role in all of this. Psychoanalysis is no universal panacea. It promotes an understanding of what has happened, but it can't *change* what has happened. If the early experiences have been too dreadful, they remain in later times as responses which are hardwired within us.

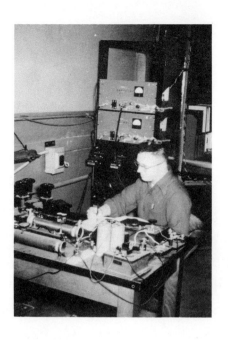

The author is shown in his third floor physics laboratory office.

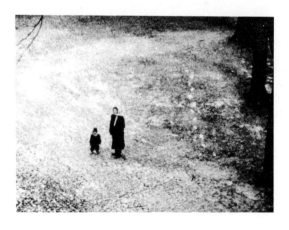

Anne and our two-year-old son are viewed from the office window.

The Second Childbirth Story

The Ecstasy

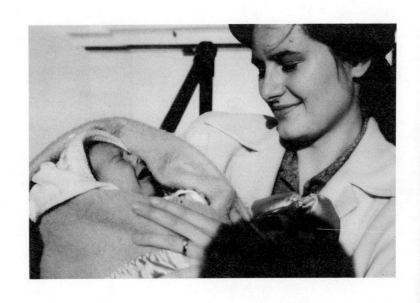

*This picture shows Anne with our second son
at his christening. He was five weeks old.*

The Second Birth: Heaven's Gift

The Professor of Obstetrics who had administered to Anne during her first childbirth was right in one sense: women are incredibly tough, even if you smash them apart. One would think that Anne, after her first childbirth experience, would not dare go through another one. But she did. And she didn't tell me until it was all over that she had gone into it with the firm expectation that she was willing to die, if that's what was required. But, she added, it was just this attitude of allowing Nature to have Her own way that, in the end, led to the knowledge that childbirth is meant to be a fulfilling experience.

This second childbirth experience was radically different from the first one, and it culminated in a manner which both astounded and delighted Anne. An event occurred that she could never have anticipated. In fact, this marvelous culmination forms the main content of the second childbirth story.

While I was still finishing graduate school, Anne became pregnant again. This was two years after the birth of our first child. In this pregnancy, as in the first, she sailed through without any pre-natal complications. She retained all of the troubles that I have described above, but they did not seem to affect the way she carried the baby.

The baby was scheduled to arrive two weeks after we had moved to my new job location, far from the Midwest. As it turned out, the baby arrived four weeks later. The baby wasn't late by a month. We were just a month off in our starting time. The extra month was helpful, because it gave us time to meet a few people and get settled. For the first few weeks, until we could rent a house, we lived in a motel with our two-year-old son. As it turned out, the family in the next unit had also come from the Midwest, and the husband was an engineer who was going to work at the same place I was. We quickly became close friends, and this friendship has continued through the years. When Anne had her second child, we left our son with them.

Our new doctor was an obstetrician who had been recommended to us, and he practiced at an excellent private hospital. This hospital was located in a university town, but was not connected to the university. The only obstetrical business here was that of delivering babies, and not of trying to train new medical students at the same time. This was exactly the type of hospital we wanted! The twin tasks of treating patients and training students are not always compatible activities, at least from the standpoint of the patient. If *The First Childbirth Story* hasn't convinced the reader of that, nothing will.

When the day came for the birth of our second child, we waved good-bye to our son and our newly-acquired friends, and went off to the hospital. I am sure that both of us were scared. After what had happened the first time, how could we feel otherwise?

There is an interesting side note here. In my new job, one of my co-workers had a wife who was also expecting. Unbeknown to us, he and his wife entered this same hospital a few hours before we did. A few minutes after they had cleared out of their assigned labor room, we arrived and moved into this same room. They had an uneventful childbirth, but with a somewhat different conclusion, I suspect, than ours.

We checked into the hospital around eleven in the evening. This hospital was not as overwhelming in scope as the massive teaching hospital we had been in the first time, but it was still a rather large hospital. Anne went into the labor room and was prepped for the delivery. I was then admitted to the room with her. The room had a pleasant atmosphere. Instead of a glaring clinical overhead light, as in the University Hospital, this room had soft reflected light from a fixture placed low on the wall at the side of the bed. The bed was a conventional type, without rails, and it was cozily positioned in a kind of nook at one end of the room. Anne can still draw a picture of exactly how the room was laid out. This isn't surprising, because she used this same room for her third childbirth, twelve years later.

In this second childbirth, Anne had the handicap of the memory of her first experience. But she also had some definite advantages. Her birth canal, having once yielded to the passage of a baby, could yield a second time more easily. Of equal importance was the fact that this time Anne was not totally fatigued as she went into serious labor. She did not have the sleep deprivation, the physical exhaustion, and the food and water deficiencies that had plagued her first childbirth. She was assured that medication was available if and when she needed it. And, finally, she had some idea of what to expect. Anne didn't bring along a cribbage board. And her mental state was quite different this time. Uppermost in her mind was one very clear idea—that she could in no way contribute to the baby's birth. This baby was going to do the job itself as Nature intended. She was firmly determined not to interfere by imposing any well-intentioned breathing exercises or relaxation techniques.

Things went completely differently this time than the last. The total time we spent in the labor room was about four hours. The contractions did their job in an efficient manner, and Anne did not have to worry about whether or not she was making progress. The contractions were painful, but not unbearable. She accepted a single injection of Demerol. When the nurse came in later to see if she needed a follow-up shot, Anne refused. Turning to the wall, she said, "Just leave me alone and I will manage." She did!

I was with Anne throughout her second labor, but just as a companion. My duties as an amateur backrubber were not requested. I could see that the contractions commanded all of Anne's attention. She was feeling serious discomfort. But she did not cry out or throw herself around on the bed. Mostly she was huddled up on her side, just letting things happen. With this attitude, she was able to keep control of herself and stay "on top" of the situation. Her contractions came one at a time, and did not overwhelm her as they had during her first childbirth. Expecting the worst, she must have been relieved that her second childbirth was manageable. I certainly was.

When the doctor finally announced that Anne was ready for the delivery room, at about four in the morning, he said I could stand outside of the delivery room door, but I could not go in. After I bade Anne good luck, they wheeled her in on the gurney, and the door closed behind them. It is possible that the doctor wouldn't have minded if I had opened the door a crack and peeked in. But I didn't, and thereby missed out on witnessing one of Nature's most unique and awe-inspiring events.

A short time later the door was opened, and I could see the doctor holding aloft a healthy seven and a half pound baby boy. Anne's arms were still strapped down to the delivery table, and she was smiling from ear to ear. After the debacle of the first childbirth, I was vastly relieved to have things turn out so well. The nurse came out of the delivery room a few minutes later, and she was shaking her head from side to side in wonder. She told me that it was a most unusual delivery. She did not explain what she meant.

It wasn't until the next day that Anne explained to me what had happened in the delivery room. This obstetrician did not use a saddle block. He understood that Anne desired a natural childbirth. Thus Anne was not numbed from the waist down, as she had been the first time. After Anne had been placed on the delivery table, her arms were strapped down and her legs were fastened into "stirrups," as was customary at that time. The baby was born a short time later. Anne said that as the baby started to come out, her hips rose instinctively and her back arched as high as possible. At least that is how it *felt*. What followed next was an experience that is best described in Anne's own words.

She felt herself stretched out on her back along the narrow rim of a large eight-foot wheel that extended down into the floor, and which turned slowly underneath her. Her head was thrown back, hanging down along the curve of the rim, her mouth open in pure abandon. The voluptuous sensations spilled over her and increased with the turnings of the wheel. The doctor called out her name and asked her to look into the mirror that had been strategically placed for her to witness the birth. She replied with difficulty, "I cannot. It is too much!" She made an effort to lift her head, but it fell back again in ecstasy.

Days later, Anne was still smiling to herself.

This mystical description of Anne's orgasmic childbirth is her reporting, not mine. I wasn't even there—I was standing outside of the closed door. At first glance, it may seem to be a fanciful allegory, but it is much more than that. Her description of it was first told to me forty years ago, and she tells it exactly the same way today. The joyous abandon that her body experienced was very real. Anne said it was the most elevating experience she could ever imagine. Time seemed to suspend itself in the pleasure of the moment. To Anne, the wheel was real—so real that she remembers wondering how such a large wheel could fit into the room. After considering the distance from her body to the floor, she reasoned that the wheel had to extend down into the floor. Then, as she marveled over this detail, the explanation presented new problems—how can a wheel turn in the floor? It appears that her brain was struggling to account for this impossible scenario, even as her feelings at that moment had the upper hand.

Today, Anne surmises that the narrow rim of the wheel she felt underneath her suggests that her spinal column was the carrier of the sensations. The eight foot diameter of the wheel, which is a size she unhesitatingly specified, approximates the arc her spine assumed as she raised up her hips, arched her back, and threw back her head. The stimulation she received by the turning of the wheel underneath her corresponds to the excitation in her pelvis produced by the slowly-emerging baby, whose head does in fact turn as its body is coming out. This turning motion of the baby's body, with its consequent stimulation of the birth canal, gave rise to pleasure signals which were then transmitted from her pelvis through the length of her spine to her brain.

But Anne has another explanation. Though she has a deep respect for scientific analyses of material phenomena, she does not believe that a rational accounting covers everything. It does not explain joy, or love, or the irrational desire to sacrifice oneself. For her, childbirth is a means of getting in touch with the mystery of life. Involving ourselves in higher-level experiences requires surrendering ourselves to the unknown. There is no doubt in her mind whatsoever that her acceptance of the possibility of death during childbirth was the core psychological ingredient in what she believes was a cosmic experience.

Several years afterward, during her psychoanalysis, Anne discussed this incident with her analyst. He told her that many doctors know this experience can occur during childbirth, but they don't like it. They feel it gets in the way of their job in delivering the baby. They prefer to be in control. It is safer, and it takes less time.

Our new baby son was brought to Anne the same day she delivered, and she immediately offered him her breast. Later on, several nurses in charge of the newborn babies came in to see the mother who had supplied six full ounces of milk to a baby in a single feeding. Anne's impression is that it was a hospital record.

After the terrible ordeal that Anne had undergone in her first childbirth, the glorious ending to her second childbirth seemed like some kind of heavenly retribution. Unfortunately, this marvelous result did not undo the damage she had incurred in her first experience. Her problems persisted, which was the reason that she later started into psychoanalysis. But at least this second childbirth did not compound the problem. It gave her, and me, an appreciation of the fact that childbirth does not have to be a disaster, and, in fact, can be a glorious experience. Childbearing seemed to Anne to be the most beautiful part of being a woman. Child rearing became for her the most important work in her life.

The Next Ten Years

Raising one child is a lot of work. Raising two is even more. I was busy at my new job, my first employment since finishing my Ph.D. in physics. Anne struggled as hard as she could to accommodate to a new rented house, new neighbors, two active young boys, and no relatives within a thousand miles. She nursed our second son for six months, until he was ready to take milk from a bottle or cup. But Anne was always tired, unable to sleep well, dependent on sleeping pills for survival. Once, when she was changing the baby in the middle of the night and was groggy from medication, her mind lapsed as she was reaching for a diaper, and he fell off the changing table onto the floor. Fortunately, he was not injured, but Anne never forgave herself for that.

Because Anne's health continued to be poor, we obtained the services of an excellent internist. He checked Anne over thoroughly and could find nothing obviously wrong with her physically, although she certainly wasn't up to par in her ability to cope with things. He referred her to a Freudian psychoanalyst, and thus got her started in a treatment program that was to last altogether for more than a decade. It is not easy to assess the effectiveness of such a program, since history does not disclose its alternatives. But the psychoanalyst had one rule that must be regarded as a definite plus: *no drugs*. Anne had taken (minimum dose) sleeping pills for so long that she had completely lost faith in her ability to fall asleep on her own. In addition, the analyst required that she must undertake to drive herself to her appointments, which were forty miles away. This was an essential step in restoring her self-confidence. During the course of Anne's psychoanalysis, the details of her first childbirth were gone over many times. This is supposed to be therapeutic, and it probably is. But it is no magic bullet for eliminating the wreckage of such an experience. Anne never returned to using sleeping pills, but she has never recovered her ability to sleep at will. Each night she still battles the prospect of sleeplessness.

Having more children seemed out of the question. We had all we could manage with two. Furthermore, the task of driving two hours a day, four days a week, to see the analyst was a job in itself for Anne. Each visit took her almost half a day to accomplish. This psychiatric treatment was not covered by insurance, and I soon found myself holding down two jobs to pay for all of the medical bills. I eventually underwent a psychoanalysis myself, and it is fair to say that the task of participating in analysis and paying for it dominated our lives for the better part of two decades. Anne was not in a position to resume her work as an interior decorator, and she never worked in that profession again.

One thing, however, had not been stamped out of Anne during all of this turmoil: her driving ambition to complete her college education. After our two boys were in school, and with the encouragement of her analyst, she enrolled as an art major at a nearby university. Her required courses did not fit in with her earlier studies, so she had to start as a lower-division student. She could only take a part-time load, so it required four years for her to finish her degree. The schoolwork was a terrible struggle for her and, indeed, for the whole family. In spite of her problems, she finally achieved her goal, a Bachelor of Arts degree. And, to her complete surprise, she received a Phi Beta Kappa key for outstanding scholarship. Anne was now thirty seven years old.

The Third Childbirth Story

The Miracle

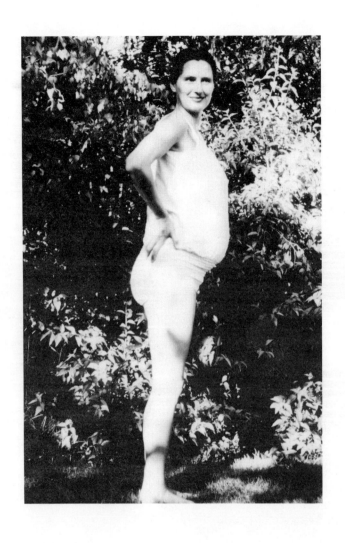

Anne, almost forty years old, is shown here in her "stretchable" bathing suit, one week before the birth of our last child. She still swam laps every day.

The Final Pregnancy

Anne decided to continue on and work for a master's degree in art, which took two more years to complete. When we were first married, Anne and I had assumed, along with most of our friends, that we would all have several children. Several generally meant more than two. But with all of the turmoil we had been through, two seemed to be a full plate. However, on Anne's thirty-ninth birthday, we discussed the fact that we had never had the daughter we someday hoped to have. Seven months later Anne completed her master's degree. Our young sons and I proudly attended her graduation ceremony, in which Anne wore the traditional black robe and black mortar board hat. Her flowing robes concealed the fact that she was seven months pregnant.

The Miracle: Freedom from Pain

Anne had been in the city for a late afternoon appointment with her analyst. After she arrived home and prepared dinner, she announced to us that she thought the baby was on the way. She reported having contractions as she drove home. It was now two months after Anne's graduation, so it was indeed time for the birth. Our two boys were fourteen and eleven years old, and well able to fend for themselves. The boys helped monitor the "pains," and, after a light dinner, Anne packed a small suitcase. She and I then took off for the same hospital in which she had delivered our second son. We arrived there in the middle of the evening, and Anne was assigned to the same labor room she had occupied almost twelve years earlier. The times had now progressed to the point where husbands were admitted to both the labor room and the delivery room. But such amenities as birthing centers were still a thing of the future.

Anne's pregnancy, like the previous ones, had been entirely normal and free of complications. She had a large bulging abdomen, but otherwise had gained no excess weight. In fact, she swam laps in our neighborhood pool right up to the morning of the day of her labor.

It had been so long since our second son was born that we had pretty much forgotten just how things were carried out in the hospital. I left the labor room while the nurse prepped Anne for the delivery, which consisted mainly in carefully shaving off the hair in the pubic area. The labor ward was empty except for us, and the nurse in the hall was the only one who seemed to be on duty in that area of the hospital. The obstetrician was nowhere to be seen. It was now late in the evening, and the whole hospital was very quiet.

Anne's contractions were coming at a steady pace, but were not yet too uncomfortable. I was beside her bed in the labor room, and we were all alone, just the two of us. Anne was lying on her back, with her knees up. The pain from the contracting uterus was felt not only in her abdomen, but also in her lower back and in her legs. She asked me to massage the inner sides of her thighs, as this region seemed to be the most spastic. I massaged the long muscles inside her thighs as she requested, but then very gently continued on to her vulva. The effect was startling! This gentle stimulation evidently triggered the release of endorphins in her brain, and the pain signals were masked over and greatly diminished. The contraction concluded with no undue feeling of discomfort. We were both greatly surprised. With each succeeding contraction I repeated this strategy, and it worked perfectly!

The Third Childbirth Story

We continued on with our new discovery for the next two hours, and it worked every time. Finally the nurse on duty came into the room to see how things were going. While she was there, Anne had another contraction. We were reluctant to carry out our intimate massage in front of the nurse, so Anne went through "this one" without the benefit of our self-designated "endorphin massage therapy." As the contraction hit its peak, Anne cried out, and at the same time quickly reached up with both hands for the bars at the head of the bedframe. Something about the way she reached up surprised me. The movement seemed to be instinctive, reflexive. It was as if she had done this same thing many times before. Yet I had never seen her do such a thing. It was almost thirty years later, during my discussions with Anne about the present book, when I finally found out that Anne had indeed, during her first childbirth, carried out this same instinctive action a great many times!

Anne's uterus was now contracting quite vigorously, but since her labor still seemed to be in its early stages, and since Anne was not complaining about any undue discomfort, the nurse made no suggestion about administering pain medication. As it turned out, none was ever needed!

After the nurse left the room, we resumed our new-found EMT pain-controlling technique. Again it worked perfectly. As long as the endorphins were stimulated, the brain did not interpret the nerve impulses from the uterus as pain signals. Anne lay comfortably on the bed, with no sign that she was ever in any serious discomfort. We continued on in this manner for another two hours. Finally the nurse appeared again. Since she had heard nothing at all from our room, she hadn't intruded on us during those two hours. But now it was time to make another check on Anne's progress. She lifted Anne's hospital gown and peered under. "Oh, my God," she exclaimed, "You're ready to deliver!" She went running out of the room to summon the obstetrician.

I was hurriedly given a surgical gown to put on, and I was allowed to join Anne after she had been put in position on the table in the delivery room. I was very excited to be in there. Finally, fourteen years after the birth of my first son, I was going to see my own baby being born! I was seated at Anne's feet, close to the left-hand side of the doctor. In my excitement, I reached out and accidentally touched Anne's thigh. This was supposed to be a sterile field, and the nurse wiped it clean. Because my hands instinctively wanted to help, I did it a second time, and then a third. Each time the nurse patiently swabbed off the area. I was beginning to see why doctors might be reluctant to have husbands in the delivery room. I appreciated the fact that no one scolded me.

The anesthesiologist was positioned just above Anne's head. He asked if she wanted a whiff of gas. Anne said: "No, but I'm thirsty." He proceeded to wet a towel, which he then wrung out so as to allow the water to trickle into her mouth while she was doing the work of pushing (her arms were strapped to the table). Anne never did accept any gas. She went through this entire childbirth without any medication except the local anesthetic for the episiotomy.

As the baby started to emerge, it was difficult for me to restrain my hands. Anne told me later that it was funny to see me partially rise out of my chair repeatedly in an effort to "assist" the process. The baby came out quickly. As the doctor raised the baby up to show Anne, his hand had hold of its thigh. Anne looked down, saw his thumb between the baby's legs, and exclaimed with a trace of disappoint: "Oh, its another boy."

"No," the doctor replied, "It's a girl!" Anne's dearest wish had been fulfilled!

At the moment the baby was beginning to come out, Anne's hips started to rise and her back began to arch, as had happened the last time. But this was not the same doctor. It was the doctor's associate. He told her firmly to keep her back flat. Anne was disappointed, but she obeyed at once. Since the doctor had inhibited her body's natural inclination to move, Anne did not experience the cosmic-oneness which had accompanied her previous childbirth. Instead, her main satisfaction this time came from the miracle of the physical event itself. Anne and I were together, as parents should be. And, of course, she was satisfied with the painfree *miracle* that had occurred in the labor room. She said it felt rewarding to do a good job—she had a glow of accomplishment. There was a sense of victory, because the task of labor and delivery did not rob her of the precious energy she needed to fully enjoy her new daughter.

Anne was almost smug about having produced a girl. She felt in a way that this was a special gift to me, because she had always thought I was deprived in my youth by not having a sister. I know my mother had always longed for a daughter. In truth, I can remember many times in the years after our two sons were born when I used to wonder what a daughter of Anne's and mine would look like. We were both very satisfied!

Where do We Go from Here?

After her third childbirth, neither Anne or I said anything to the doctor about our spectacularly successful "endorphin massage therapy." This is an intimate subject, and not one that is easy to discuss openly. Also, it is not a procedure that would logically fit into the standard methods of medical practice. But this story should be told to someone, somewhere. Almost thirty years have passed since our daughter was born, and we have revealed our secret to no one, not even to our two daughters-in-law, who have each produced two grandchildren. The new babies born in the last thirty years number in the billions. Perhaps some of these mothers could have profited from our experience.

The story of the stroke that Anne suffered during her first childbirth has never been revealed to anyone, except to some of her doctors. How often does such a tragedy occur? Countless stories have been written about women who were never quite the same again after childbirth. Could they have suffered a similar fate? Can such a fate be prevented? The medical practices that are carried out during childbirth were formulated mainly by male doctors, and male doctors are notoriously lacking in direct birth experience. Men are undoubtedly good technicians in handling the medical procedures of childbirth, but they may not have a proper appreciation of the emotional factors involved. Indeed, the chauvinistic attitude which still prevails today among many physicians is that women are by nature very emotional, and many of their supposed illnesses are in fact just products of their lively imaginations.

As a physicist, I have spent my life in research. One of the main tasks of a research scientist is to ascertain whether what seems to be a new discovery is in reality genuine, or whether it was just an accidental result. The key to verifying this discovery is *reproducibility*. Can other workers reproduce this result? Seen in this perspective, what did Anne and I establish in our unexpected venture into painless childbirth?

There is no question that the result we achieved was genuine. When Anne received a very mild sexual stimulation, the contraction did not hurt. When she did not receive this soothing stimulation, the contraction was very painful. The scientific basis for this phenomenon is well-known and well-understood. Sexual stimulation releases endorphins in the brain, and these endorphins alter the perception of pain. Endorphins, like morphine, belong to the opium family of pain killers. Soldiers in combat and athletes in sports sometimes incur injuries which, at the time, are completely disregarded. The participants in these activities are in mental states that, while not overtly sexual in nature, are at a very high emotional level. T. E. Lawrence, the famous Lawrence of Arabia, wrote in his book *Seven Pillars of Wisdom* about the problem of bearing up under torture. As he stated the matter, what you must do is get yourself into a state where you can interpret the pain they are inflicting on you as sexual. The pain then recedes to a level you can tolerate. But you must be careful not to let on to your tormentors that this has taken place. Otherwise, they will sense what has happened, and will take appropriate countermeasures.

The capacity of the human brain to alter the perception of pain is truly phenomenal. When I was a sailor in uniform in World War II, I had the opportunity to appear on stage in a theater as an assistant for a well-known magician. He was performing a demonstration of hypnosis for the audience. He told one of my fellow sailors, who had been hypnotized, to hold out his arm with the palm down. Then he lit a match, told the hypnotized sailor that he would feel no pain, and briefly held the lighted match under the sailor's outstretched palm. I was standing three feet away, and I could see that the sailor never flinched: he felt nothing! The magician was not a medical man, but he understood, better than some physicians, the power of the spoken voice to alleviate pain by suggestion alone.

The problem with Anne's and my discovery is that we have had no opportunity to repeat it. We did not have another child. And we have not asked anyone else to try and repeat it. This may be a difficult technique to work with, for several reasons. The procedure itself is a very intimate one that cannot be performed by just anyone, or just anywhere. The stimulation must be sufficient to do the job, and yet subtle or gentle enough that it can be maintained over a prolonged period of time. And it might not be the type of thing that doctors would want to put into their textbooks. What happens if it stops working? What happens if outside disturbances intervene? What happens if no husband is available? It is possible that this sexual stimulation during labor is in fact a technique which the husband can easily administer to his expecting wife, once he has been informed about it. But it is also possible that Anne and I were incredibly lucky, with just the right circumstances to make it work. Because childbirth is a universal experience, and the problems associated with it are so real, research along these lines would seem to be a worthwhile endeavor. Since only natural forces are being employed, it is hard to see where such an attempt could bring harm to anyone.

The End of the Story

With the birth of our third child, Anne's childbearing years drew to a close. Hence our story about Anne's childbirths logically ends here. But it is of interest to continue the tale a little farther.

Anne breast fed our new baby daughter for as long as the baby wanted to nurse. I still clearly remember, nineteen months after the birth, seeing Anne walk down the hall toward me in the middle of the afternoon, her cheeks wet with tears. "She doesn't want the breast any more," Anne exclaimed. Her feelings were a mixture of joy and sadness. She was happy that our baby daughter had successfully passed from one developmental phase to the next, but she was sorry to close one of the most intimate and satisfying chapters in her role as a mother.

Anne and I are now approaching our allotted three-score and ten years. The three childbirth stories we have shared here with our readers happened so long ago that they seem to us like ancient history. But they were so significant that they continue to retain a real vitality in our memories.

The torch has been passed to the next generation. Our two sons are grown up, married, and have families—the oldest has two girls, and his brother has two boys. In fact, as I am writing these words today, our oldest grandchild, a granddaughter, is celebrating her tenth birthday. Our own daughter, who is much younger than her brothers, is still a free spirit.

Looking back, there is remarkably little communication between generations on the topic of childbirth. Anne once asked her mother about her childbirth experiences, and her mother replied that she held a holy picture in her hand during labor. She had her babies at home. The only detail I learned about my own birth was that the delivery was held up for an hour so the obstetrician could finish her dinner. My Canadian grandmother told me that when she had her children, back in the 1800's, the doctor came to the house to deliver them, and he charged her five dollars each time.

Appropriately, our daughters-in-law consulted medical people of their own generation when they were preparing to become mothers. Had this book been available, would they have benefited? In her desire to help, Anne emphasized to both mothers-to-be that birth was a joyous occasion—but that was all she said. Some topics just do not lend themselves to easy conversation.

The childbirth experience, with its initial pain, its final sense of fulfillment in the birth of a child, and the bond that it makes between husband and wife, stands as an encapsulation of the process we call *life*. Hopefully, the three Childbirth Stories told here will in some manner serve to deepen and enrich this experience for expectant couples, and maybe even stand as a bridge between the generations.

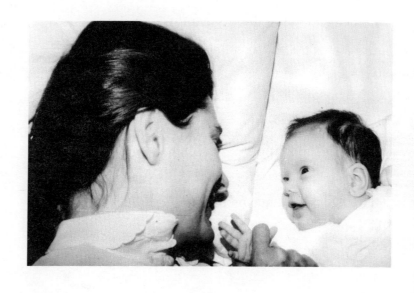

Anne and our two-month old daughter are having a conversation.

In Conclusion

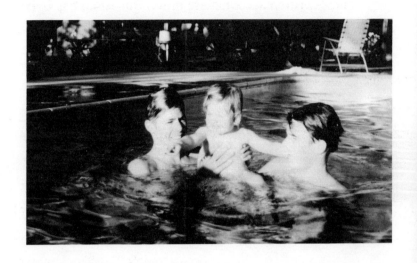

Our three children, at ages sixteen, two,
and thirteen, are taking a swim together.

Some Final Thoughts

These written accounts are mine. But Anne has lived them, so she has a better understanding of the scope of her sufferings during her first childbirth, and of the significance of the benefits she reaped in her later childbirths. Are her experiences relevant to other mothers-to-be? Childbirth itself is universal. Though women vary in disposition from person to person, yet in their psychological makeup, just as in their physical anatomy, they all possess the same basic emotional mechanisms for dealing with the pangs of childbirth. The stories I have related here seem to be outside of most people's common experience (although similar stories are undoubtedly known to others). Allowing for the differences in couples, I believe these stories may be of some benefit to those who find themselves in a similar situation. If I don't write them down and attempt to publish them, they will be lost. Indeed, they have in a sense been lost for the past thirty years. The events I have described here are as accurate as I can make them, down to the last detail. It is my sincere intention to pass on any useful information that can be extracted from our experiences—the tragic, the sublime, and the victorious. Although I don't recall every detail (after all, I am going back more than forty years for the first of these stories), the things I have written here are things that I *do* remember, or that Anne remembers. I didn't make up anything, apart from my sojourns into the mind of the Professor, and these passages are well identified in the text.

The Professor who figured so prominently in the first story has been dead for many years. He was in fact a sincere, conscientious doctor, and I know that he was held in the highest regard by his students, some of whom are my personal friends. If he could read the story about himself that I have written here, I think he would be genuinely appalled. I don't think he had a clue as to the negative consequences of what he considered to be good teaching practices.

I believe it was Nietzsche who said, "The things that don't kill us make us stronger." This statement is only partly true. A broken leg doesn't kill us, but the healed leg often does not have its original strength. Physical blows, over the long haul, weaken us. But physical blows can toughen the spirit. Anne was, and is, a fighter. Things never came easily for her. She set her own course, and, to the best of her ability, she has carried it through. Anne is the most self-disciplined person I have ever met. She still suffers from the maladies of the past, but she follows an undeviating program of physical exercises, and every day she works at her tasks as an artist, writer and homemaker from morning to night. In addition to helping raise grandchildren, she has also found time to assist a surprising number of other people, especially young people, in various ways. Maybe the old Professor was right after all with his message, at least as stated in my fanciful reconstruction, that women are indeed incredibly tough.

There is one more message here, which has to do with the role of fathers in the childbirth process. This role has of course changed remarkably in the past forty years, in the sense that hospitals now allow the father to participate almost as much as he wishes to. After our first child was born, I had a complex set of reactions. My first reaction was one of elation for the birth of a fine son. My next was a feeling of dismay when I found out what

Anne had been through in the last phases of her childbirth. This feeling deepened in the succeeding months as it became apparent how much damage had been done, and it was accompanied by another feeling, a sense of guilt—I had impregnated Anne and caused all of this, but she was the one who had to suffer. As a final reaction, there developed a sense of nameless anger at having been excluded from the birth process. This was my wife's and my child, and I should have somehow been allowed to be a participant. Of course, if I had actually been in the labor room with Anne when she was in her final hours of torment, I might not have been able to handle it. The Professor might have had two patients on his hands instead of one. Under conditions as they were then, perhaps I wouldn't have been of much help to Anne. She needed someone who could speak to her with authority and reassure her that she was going to survive. Authority requires experience. Nevertheless, I was offended at not having been allowed to be present at that crucial time. If I had been there, I told myself, I might have at least prevented the Professor from carrying out his merciless training exercise (which he never did acknowledge to us had taken place). I might have held Anne's hand when she most needed it!

In the second childbirth, I was allowed to be with Anne in the labor room, and then, later, I was permitted to stand outside of the delivery room door. In the third childbirth, many years later, I was allowed full access to the event. So things have improved. It is in the first childbirth where the husband's role may be most crucial. Second and third childbirths are usually easier than the first, if there are no complications. This of course is well known. Many training classes now exist expressly for first-time parents. The husband is more qualified than anyone else to furnish the emotional support that a laboring mother requires, as Dr. Grantly Dick-Read recognized early on. And the sense of sharing that a husband and wife obtain during this difficult time serves to bond them together in a very real sense. Being a part of the birth process makes the husband realize more than anything else what it means to become a *father*.

The real tragedy of Anne's first childbirth was that the Professor did not recognize the importance of the emotional factors involved. *The First Childbirth Story*

In Conclusion

hopefully helps to highlight the necessity of providing this emotional support. *The Third Childbirth Story* demonstrates that husbands in the labor room may, under the right circumstances, be more than just bystanders. And *The Second Childbirth Story* shows that, given the proper situation, mothers may receive Nature's sublime affirmation of their status in the eternal scheme of things. Without mothers, there would be no story at all.

More About Ourselves

For our faithful readers who have followed this story of Anne's childbirth experiences to its very end, I have a confession to make. As you may have noticed in these tales, only two Proper Names ever appear: the name J. Cameron, which is on the cover and title page, and the name Anne, which occurs throughout the book. These are not our real names. After considerable soul-searching and consultation with family, we felt it was better for all concerned that we remain anonymous. Although these stories happened a long time ago, there are still people living, including in particular our own children, who are involved with these events. However, apart from the use of fictitious names, everything else is real. My wife and I actually hold the degrees that have been attributed to us, we attended universities in the manner described, the family genealogies are accurate, the pictures are of us and our children, and the myriad events that have been described here all happened. I did not "wallpaper" these stories. My aim in this book was to entertain, in the sincerest form of this verb, and hopefully to instruct. The first story was, and still is, a very painful one, but my purpose in telling it was not to assess blame. Pain, unfortunately, is a part of life, whether we like it or not. And it is not shared equally among us. The main virtue in the first story, as I would like to think of it, is that it serves to make the last two stories more credible. These last two vignettes, brief as they are, tell of truly remarkable events. They are the stories that can be built on—that can lead to deeper discoveries in the mystery known to us only as the *human experience.*

Finally, I would like to thank the person I have called Anne for sharing her life, her sufferings, and her joys with me. Men are given to have certain experiences in life, and women are given to have other, quite different, experiences. When a man and a woman are joined together in holy matrimony, they share these experiences, and each of them is the richer for it. This lady known to you only as Anne has done everything within her power to contribute to the betterment of her husband and children, and I hope that I have done the same for her. Neither of us is perfect, of course, but life itself is not perfect. It was never intended to be that way.

The Medical Records

After this manuscript had been completed and sent out to a few selected reviewers, I started wondering if the medical records of these childbirths might still exist. These would fill out the stories presented here, which are based on memories from many years ago. It turned out that the medical records of the first childbirth do in fact exist in the archives of the University Hospital, but the medical records of the second and third childbirths, which were at a different hospital, were destroyed when the children each reached their eighteenth birthday. After considerable searching, the records of the first childbirth were finally located on an old spool of microfilm and were copied and sent to us.

Anne (I will still call her by that name here) did not want to, and has not, looked at these hospital records. This is a task I assigned to myself, although these are, properly speaking, her records. Anne had to personally request them from the hospital. The hospital will send them out to no one else.

In Conclusion

It was with some trepidation and with a feeling of awe that I opened the thick envelope containing the medical records of Anne's first childbirth. Here was the past coming back to speak to us. These records are almost half a century old! What would they say? Would they substantiate our memories? The first thing I saw was the street address of our student apartment. It doesn't seem possible that we moved away from there more than forty years ago. The recollections it evoked were overpowering. We lived there for the first four years of our marriage. Our past is really our most precious asset, painful though it may be in places.

I rapidly read through the records to find out two things: are they informative, and do they agree with the facts we set forth in *The First Childbirth Story?* The first question was quickly answered. The records are indeed very informative. In particular, they contain detailed comments made by the attending physicians during the course of Anne's long labor, the kinds of comments that a patient normally never sees—at least in my experience. The second question was also quickly answered, but not in quite the way I expected. Most of the facts in *The First*

Childbirth Story turned out to be very accurate—our memories are good. But the first part of the story, the time when we entered the hospital, is incorrect. Anne did indeed start her long labor on a Wednesday morning, as stated in the story. And she did go for three days and two nights with continuous contractions and essentially no sleep, as also stated in the story. This is the way we both remember it. But she spent the first day of her labor (or near-labor) at home—not in the hospital. It wasn't until late that night when we went to the hospital, which is *not* the way we remembered it. The events that took place after we once entered the hospital accurately follow the time sequence we have given here. This discrepancy raised a problem for me as an author. My first thought was to simply rewrite the first part of *The First Childbirth Story* so as to agree with this new information. But this would be a fiction. I obviously don't remember the details of exactly what happened that first Wednesday, so I would have to make up something. And this is not supposed to be a fictional story. I finally decided to leave the original story alone. The essential elements as given there are correct. The feelings we had at the time—our optimism, which turned into dismay as the hours dragged on with no progress being made—are accurately portrayed in the narrative as I first wrote it down. This account of events is more true-to-life than any technically-correct modification I could at this point make up. The main difference made in the story by our late entry into the hospital was that Anne and I actually played our first game of cribbage in the hospital on a Thursday morning, and not on a Wednesday morning as stated in the story. The important fact is that she won the game, not the exact time it was played. The *really* significant fact, of course, is that we played cribbage at all during her labor.

The medical records presented another problem to me as an author. Do I include them as a part of this book? Again, my first thought was to add them in as a part of the written manuscript. With the aid of modern copying equipment, I could include some really crucial comments made by the Professor of Obstetrics, displayed as actually set forth in his own handwriting. But, aided in part by some strong advice from my wife, who—as I stated above—has not looked at these records, I finally decided against this course of action. The records add to the details, but they do not change the human drama.

In spite of the informative nature of the medical records for Anne's first childbirth, they lack one piece of information that I had thought might be there. The account of exactly what happened when Anne reached her point of crisis during her second stage of labor is missing. The rest of the hour-to-hour report of her labor is succinctly and compellingly set forth in a two-page Labor Sheet that forms the core of these records. The Labor Sheet is the detailed description of the labor, and the information it contains is of two types. The first is a factual accounting of the measurements taken to record the progress of the labor, and it includes the medical procedures that were carried out. The second is a *commentary* by the attending physicians as to Anne's physical and emotional condition. The factual entries include items such as the time of day, the degree of dilation, the frequency and strength of the contractions, the orientation of the baby's head, Anne's blood pressure, and the various medications that were administered. The commentary includes remarks such as how much sleep Anne was getting, and how she seemed to be holding up—or not holding up—under the ordeal of the labor. It is concise and surprisingly graphic as it describes Anne's physical and emotional deterioration during the slow progress of her long labor. As Anne's labor approached its crucial final hours, the commentary becomes more comprehensive. But then, just at the point where the records should fill in the details of Anne's time of crisis, the commentary as to her condition abruptly stops; it is never resumed. From this point on, just the factual data on the progress of her labor is entered into the Labor Sheet

The last two detailed commentaries shown on Anne's Labor Sheet were written by the Professor of Obstetrics himself. The first of these was made at the time he ruptured her membranes, just before he put her to sleep with a large dose of barbiturates. The second was made two and a half hours later, at the time when Anne—groggily attempting to struggle back into consciousness—was just moving into the second stage of her labor. These final reports by the Professor accurately confirm—and in fact extend—the information I had put together in *The First Childbirth Story* with respect to Anne's physical and emotional condition just prior to her final ordeal. The time at which the Professor made his final commentary is also the official time of onset of Anne's second stage of labor. After this entry, no further information is provided in any of the hospital records as to how Anne fared during the period of her very vigorous second stage of labor. Nor is there any reference to the subsequent hour she spent in the delivery room. For this information, we have only Anne's recall.

The University Hospital records, in my opinion, substantiate the essential accuracy of the dramatic events that are related in *The First Childbirth Story*.

In the narration of the *Three True Childbirth Stories*, I am simply describing the totality of my wife's experiences, in the hope that our readers will obtain useful information from them—from the failures as well as the successes. The union of these three experiences—*The Agony, The Ecstasy,* and *The Miracle*—makes each of them more meaningful than any one of them would be if taken separately.

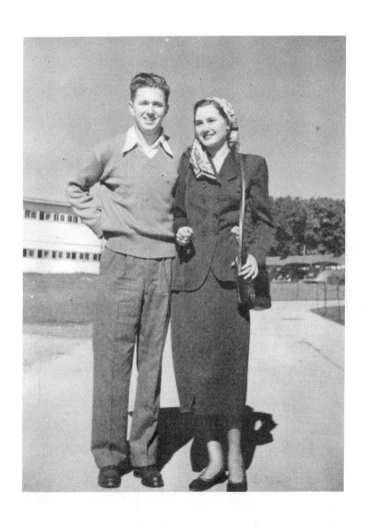

*The author and his wife-to-be are shown here
at age twenty-two, a year before their marriage.*

Order Form

POSTAL ORDER

El Mac Books

P.O. Box 3300
Livermore, CA 94550
U.S.A.

Please send me_____ copies of *The Agony; The Ecstasy; The Miracle: Three True Childbirth Stories*

> 1 - 4 copies @ $12.95 ea US, $17.95 ea Can
> 5 or more   @ $9.00 ea US, $12.50 ea Can

Sales tax 8.25% for books shipped to a California address.

Shipping book rate: $2.00 for the first book, and 50 cents for each additional book (may take three to four weeks).

Shipping priority mail and foreign mail: $3.50 for the first book, and $1.00 for each additional book (US funds).

Name_____

Address_____

City_____

State_____Zip_____

Country_____

Order Form

POSTAL ORDER

El Mac Books

P.O. Box 3300
Livermore, CA 94550
U.S.A.

Please send me_____ copies of *The Agony; The Ecstasy;*
The Miracle: Three True Childbirth Stories

     1 - 4 copies @ $12.95 ea US, $17.95 ea Can
     5 or more   @ $9.00 ea US, $12.50 ea Can

Sales tax 8.25% for books shipped to a California address.

Shipping book rate: $2.00 for the first book, and 50 cents for
each additional book (may take three to four weeks).

Shipping priority mail and foreign mail: $3.50 for the first
book, and $1.00 for each additional book (US funds).

Name_____

Address_____

City_____

State_____Zip_____

Country_____